MW01281828

MERCURY IN LEMONADE

TAMAS PANITZ

NEW SMUT SERIES
from the **NEW BOOKS** imprint

NEW SMUT SERIES is a subdivision of NEW BOOKS publishing.

NEW SMUT SERIES, NEW BOOKS, and NEW: THE
JOURNAL OF AMERICAN POETRY are all published
directly through the print-on-demand website Lulu.com. Our
titles can be purchased from the Lulu marketplace or by
contacting tamaspanitz@gmail.com

A list of our titles and links to purchase can be found on our
tumblr: www.tumblr.com/newjournalofpoetry

To advertise with us or for any other actually appealing inquires
that are in no way submissions, contact us at
NewJournalofPoetry@gmail.com

NEW PUBLICATIONS:
75360 Via Domingo
 Palm Desert, CA. 92211

ISBN 978-1-387-50631-6

List of Illustrations:

PART I

MERCURY IN LEMONADE

TAMAS PANITZ

PART I

1

It was then that a discomfort, a swaying sensation, awakened me from my reverie. I opened my eyes and instantly closed them again, plunged into a vertiginous flash of unwanted memories in which I recognized the blue velvet trousers and matching vest that I wore, with their trim of yellow rope tassels. I do not like first impressions, either to give or to receive them. These articles of clothing were fashioned for me at my request by my servant from antique curtains found in the attic of my castle. After a deep breath, I reached my fingers out above my head to the table that stands behind my couch, and there they met with the sticky wet skin of a dolma. I felt with my fingernail along the grape-leaf's edge. I began to unfold it, slowly, with great care, such that the sodden leaf remained intact as I shifted it and eventually scraped off and dropped its inner load of rice onto the plate. After some moments of feeling the leaf over and double-checking my work, I brought the grape-leaf down onto my face and spread it across my nose, smoothing it over my lower eyelids and out past my cheekbones. The cool leaf clung to me with a woody roughness and I felt suddenly aware of the roughness of my socks — which caused my toes to rub and flick convulsively against each other.

To distract myself from this discomfort, one which I knew to be for the greater part purely mental, I decided immediately to erect my penis (using both hands). This done, alleviating my irritation, I began to think of my girlfriend. I saw her on her side, with her upper leg bent at the hip and knee to form a right angle; then simultaneously with her elbow, bent, masturbating me with the crook of her arm; and thirdly, her disembodied hands at rest on the green velvet of my couch. These images brought a feeling of profound tenderness with them. My couch, a wood-framed affair that had been cut from a single immense beam of a French cathedral, exhaled the softest fragrance of Frankincense and bee pollen. You will have to bear with me, dear reader, when I say that I impulsively dragged my fish-fork up one of its legs.

This fish-fork had once belonged to a set of measuring spoons that, through careful manipulation, had gradually been transformed into various miniature items of cutlery, none of them spoons. The last remaining spoon at this moment lies on the kitchen counter some feet behind me: it is the largest — the Full Tablespoon — and I contemplate two potential lives for it. Though neither of these potential transformations is sufficiently clear as to be executed at this time, nonetheless they vie for dominance in my decision, one culinary mass pitted against the other. As my mind wanders back to the issue of the final spoon, my penis immediately softens. I no longer concern myself with it after wrapping it cursorily in a linen napkin and leaving it tucked under my shirt-front (I mean my penis).

I note that this make-shift holster or scabbard is what Latins would have called a *vagina*, which is exactly where a sword would go when it's *not* in use. One might argue from this that the sex act is the only act that is not sexual, after all, and the neurotic scattered state that spreads in an inverse relation to libidinous sexuality, its apparently endless dissimulation, is in fact so much unanticipated consummation.

2.

I dozed off, and awakened, apparently several hours later. My eyes hurt, and two cones of pain reached from my eyeballs like spotlights combing the roof of my skull. I was disturbed to discover the manner in which I'd left my penis, and brusquely slid it into my pants, fearing that my manservant or some other member of the household might have seen it; but at the same time I felt relieved of this fear by the fact that I had not been awakened, for I am a very light napper. I propped myself up on my forearms and glanced into the kitchen to satisfy myself as to the position of the measuring spoon: it had not been moved, and this would have been a sure indication of any housekeeping.

I dropped my arm to feel under the lip of the large Oriental rug that sits before my couch. I should say 'once Oriental," because this rug is made of fibers painstakingly repurposed from hundreds of ancient rugs, and rewoven into a hideous massive strip of colorful flashes and dull pools of annihilated patterns vaguely poisonous in hue.

At last my fingers, grimed from the little specks of dirt that had permeated the rug, made contact with a very heavy sheet of paper– in fact, the backing to a calendar. Once extricated, this large sheet containing various notes, dates, phone numbers, and reminders, began yielding up for me the variety of information that I needed to start my day. However, just as I was entering upon a train of thought concerning an upcoming doctor's appointment, I realized that I was hungry. In a split-second decision to have a turkey sandwich, I picked up my servant's bell from the foot of my couch, and rang it.

3.

Unfortunately, my manservant's entry to the room coincided with my ever increasing wakefulness, and I had just come to that peculiar state in which one suddenly remembers one's dream. The need to write down this particular dream was imperative. The dream was extraordinary for me, both because I never dream, and because its content was something of great value to those concerned with its theme. Therefore I was rather brusque in giving my manservant his instructions. Annoyed by the self-caused delay in my task of recording the dream, I somewhat viciously asked my man if he had seen five dollars on my nightstand. Of course, I knew him to be a paragon of honest hard work and a man of dignity — and he being used to my moods quietly assured me with something of a wry smile that he had not, and then excused himself.

Displeased with this interaction, I quickly called after him that we were friends. This of course is untrue, as I am his employer. Nonetheless, I enjoyed the ambiguity into which this phrase had hurled us, both master and servant, as it were. We were forced mentally to examine what nascent potential friendship there might have been between us, and forced to see those imaginary versions of ourselves rise up and fail before this statement of mine, incapable of meeting its terms.

At the head of my couch is a small piece of furniture containing a single drawer. The provenance of this decor is too complex to recite even to myself —suffice it to say that this item began life in a form vastly different from that in which it lives today. Without moving the main of my body, I prized open the little drawer, and groping around I secured a small notebook and several pencils that I am in the habit of keeping there, along with an eraser. I put these items in my lap and allowed a few of the pencils to roll into the crevice between my body and the sofa. All of this brought about a feeling of extraordinary contentment.

4.

I'm around six years old, at the beach, playing in the shallow wave-breaks. My mother watches me from a nearby pavilion. Suddenly it becomes overcast, the water slows, its motion and feeling become gelatinous. The waves take minutes to break, so between the slow waves I can plunge my hand with impunity into the troughs where stones are momentarily visible. I pick up one red and one grey, both covered with many miniscule heart-shaped bioluminescent carbuncles. I bring these stones to my mother who contemplates them briefly — until her attention is drawn to the sky with the rest of the beachgoers.

Sort of Kabbalistic geometrical forms pulse with light in the darkening sky. These forms stretch an enormous distance, apparently to the surface of the earth. There's no doubt we're witnessing a cosmic event, visible from much of the globe.

A dazzlingly beautiful beam of golden light descends upon the surface of the now utterly calm sea, and speeds towards the beach. Gradually, in groups of two or three or singly, this ray of light lifts individuals effortlessly into the sky and sends them zooming up towards its source. I observe one sexy beachgoer with revealing denim shorts lifted into the air above me…

It was at this point that I ejaculated in my sleep, and at this point again in my retelling, I lost a small emission. Whether or not the golden beam would have taken me did not become clear, since I immediately switched dreams, as is always the case with my nocturnal emissions. This second dream was of little interest and I do not feel tempted to record it in detail.

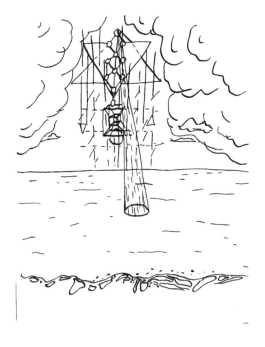

"A dazzlingly beautiful beam of golden light descends upon the surface of the now utterly calm sea, and speeds towards the beach."

The creak of the kitchen door, which connects the kitchen to the West wing of my palace, alerted me to the presence of my girlfriend.

Sure enough, I saw her pale slender fingers emerge and grasp the edge of the door. I noted her filed triangular nails, each bearing a glass gem in the middle of the nail, and told myself to remember to complement her on them. Her hand visibly flexed, and she lifted the door toward the frame so it would slide silently upon its hinges. In the gap of the passageway I saw her luminous eyes, first her eyes, and then her form, an unearthly milky white, that I found somehow evocative of her alien scent, a feeling common to brown men like myself. (There is a well-known connection between scent-attraction and genetic diversity.) With these sensations came a rush of associations that were intensely erotic. I uttered a few disconnected statements, mostly regarding the mysterious loss of my stomach hair and the value of setting our hawk-moth traps out in the morning, rather than persisting in our usual evening-time routine.

She approached me in a markedly straight line, even though that necessitated her vaulting over an ottoman, which she did so quickly and gracefully it was as if it were never done at all. This ottoman had been adapted to its current purpose from an old wooden television set, on which were drawn Raphael-esque doodles in colored chalk-paint.

Just as she neared the place where I reclined, my man entered with the turkey sandwich. My girlfriend decided then against whatever it was she had been contemplating and veered to the side, directing her steps instead to the deeply shaded patio, much overgrown with bougainvillea and jasmine and trumpet vines, where birds and bees and such kept up a continual hum.

As the French doors closed behind her the room was returned to its accustomed quiet. A small folding table was quickly erected before me, and the sandwich placed on it with some utensils, though these purely for formality. I quipped that I had not been forewarned that this would be a photo-shoot, but alas, my man, great servant that he is, had already disappeared to his duties in the rest of the house.

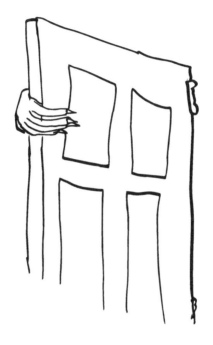

"I noted her filed triangular nails, each bearing a glass gem in the middle of the nail, and told myself to remember to complement her on them."

The grape-leaf that I had moulded to my face, now quite dry, fell from me as I sat upright. I retained this curious half-mask in the drawer at my side, lest it should be somehow crushed or disposed of without my knowledge. I felt beneath my thigh and found one of my pencils, though the lead tip had been snapped by my motion. I did not reproach myself, however, and noted that this destruction gave me pleasure and a feeling of relief, as it discharged energy from some larger chaotic force I had unconsciously felt weighing on me. I carefully placed the pencil so it was facing me under the lip of my plate. I pinched, then, such that my fingers met in the middle, my penis a few times and stopped once it began to swell. I then picked up my sandwich, but noticing my rings I replaced it on the plate. I then began removing my rings, from right to left across both hands.

Without going into unnecessary detail, these rings are in the shape of various animals, some of them ancient, others common enough — silver baubles that might be found at any outdoor market. One of them I strongly suspected to be possessed by a demon, but after certain experiments I believe the demon capable of exchanging his vessel for a neighboring one to avoid destruction.

I arranged my rings in a crescent around the turkey sandwich, such that they all faced inward and I could still easily pick up my sandwich from where I was sitting. I muttered a Sanskrit prayer whose words I knew vaguely as a dedication of my nourishment to the Buddhas, Sanghas, and various others; however, I had long ago mentally replaced these personages with The Beatles, Dogs, and Misused Chess Pieces.

I had the idea then to look back into my journal for a poem I had written a few days before, and though I was not certain of its content I recalled feeling somewhat excited about it, and sought it now with some anticipation as an aperitif to my meal.

Driving without my hair
going to the car wash, but only
to rinse off some melons
my girlfriend grew for me.
I can see her shoes smoking
as she walks toward me
through Center Square. Everything
I ever knew, I'm liquidating.
It's just me and the melons now, and we
swim like letters no literacy can pervade.

I have mixed feelings after all about this poem – or fragment, really. In some ways I'm disappointed, but it does possess a certain charm, and I'm tempted to continue it.

The next section, I decide, will be devoted to the theme of liquidation. For a second I think I will continue writing, but in the time it takes me to think it my enthusiasm for the poem has dwindled down to almost nothing.

Down in mood, I take a bite of my sandwich, and instantly regret my delay in eating it, for the bread has been made sodden by the mayonnaise, and the summer heat has made me suspect its edibility.

I worry that, if I were to eat all of the sandwich I might be too weak from battling its bacteria to join my girlfriend for sexual intercourse later, something we have both been looking forward to after her week-long absence to the city of her birth. Out of perhaps an excess of caution, I take only one more bite and content myself with the pickle and small chocolate cookie that my manservant has thoughtfully brought for me.

I consider whether to remove my rings from the plate but decide to leave them with the exception of a thumb ring designed as a bat with encircling outstretched wings: this I put on the tip of my nose, and hold it there by pressure from my upper lip. The metallic smell helps soothe my stomach and clear my mind.

My eyes focus on a very large specimen of Mexican fruit-bat preserved in a glass specimen-jar along the far wall, among other curiosities. I think I catch a gleam from the creature's eyes, as he hangs in his glass prison. My penis, I find, has absolutely no feeling at all during this interaction.

At first a mere thing of note, my communication with this very large nocturnal beast deepened, and I felt a channel of intrigue open between us, through which rushed a great deal of information. By information I mean one central idea, and along with it, in a luminous cloud, all the extrinsic matter that might be deduced from it. On the surface, this idea presented to me a vision of my girlfriend, her beautiful form, her strength, her person — but at the same time she was (in this communication) a cipher. An unrelated second tier of information flowed along with this image of my girlfriend in a kind of binary fashion, posing itself as a question. Would rigorous disassociation, the dispelling of all seemingly forgone conclusions into their ruined parts, the removal of all interactions from their usual outcomes, the wrecking of teleologies — would this discipline eventually lead to a re-association, presenting a pseudo-objectivity, like the fabulously beautiful portraits of baseball players I have seen executed by flies behind a Memphis restaurant?

I chuckled, impressed by the bat's insightfulness but also amused by his apparent lack of understanding. As if my behavior needed to justify itself with utility! The mere thought of it was condescension. Would he ask ants, bees, drugs, or ghosts what they expect from their...

I decided that he was dangerous, and to keep a closer eye on him in the future. As if turned by an invisible hand, the bat slowly rotated until it faced the wall away from me, and with his eyes hidden, all communication ceased. I soon tired of contemplating his shriveled haunches.

7.

Just then, my real girlfriend entered from the portico. She had apparently soaked a large fig-leaf and softened its fibers such that it could be molded to her features. She now wore this peculiar mask with two narrow eye-slits. She proceeded to inform me, in a very quiet voice, so I had to lean forward and cup my hand to my ear to hear it, that she had dreamt that we were broken up. Astonished, I in turn confessed that two nights ago I had been subject to that same dream, though, as I learned from her, the details differed. This was to be expected, because mine was entirely made-up.

We assured each other of our mutual love, and that neither of us had any intention of breaking off our erotic partnership. She then told me she was hungry and exited directly. I regretted not asking her what she was going to eat, and contemplated getting up to follow her, when my attention was drawn to my completely erect glans — something I had not noticed during this conversation. I reasoned that my erection had begun first with the image of my girlfriend, and was then reinforced by her actual presence, such that it had now reached the peak of arousal.

I quickly grabbed the top piece of bread from my sandwich and with a few strokes I ejaculated onto it. Then after folding it carefully in half I threw it into the wastebasket at the foot of my couch. I felt this unorthodox disposal of the bread justified for obvious reasons.

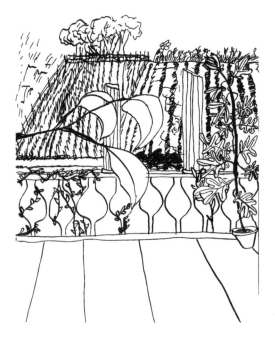

"My real girlfriend entered from the portico."

8

Now that I had finished my meal I began returning my rings to their respective fingers. As I grasped the penultimate ring, however, I immediately flung it from my hand. It was burning hot. The ring rolled onto the floor as I shook my hand vigorously to cool my damaged fingers.

The ring in question, in the design of a Dodo bird with its legs almost in its mouth, rolled a few feet across the carpet, and I felt a momentary fear that it might catch fire. However, a second, more disturbing fear stole over me, and I reached my unburnt hand out to retrieve the cursed object. As I had suspected, the Dodo was now perfectly cool to the touch, much as I wished it otherwise. It felt no different than any ring that had been sitting on a porcelain plate contemplating a sandwich: no sign of its recent temperature remained. To keep the thing in isolation would be pointless – as I have said, the demon who had just inhabited it was capable of jumping vessels and had surely already taken up a new residence.

I slid the Dodo bird onto its finger (left middle, for it was a cypher for another ring, one used by the Flamen Dialis, noble priests of Jupiter). With my burnt fingers in my mouth, I cast a glance through the french doors to the portico, and at the great flat expanse of Arkansas. Above the high rows of corn and dank lots of rice, above the mown fields with square swamps between them, I could see, by means of an extraordinarily slowed cerebral cortex (yes, read it and be amazed, scientists!), lines of telepathic intelligence zippered across the land where kudzu crouched in giant magnetic shells among strips of trees. I removed my fingers from my mouth and plunged them through the cheese of my sandwich to let them rest amid the sliced turkey, where they found total relief.

The sunlight had a crisp clear quality to it, especially after my sojourn to the dank hell of Memphis, nonsensically named for that great city that stands clitoris to the Nile; so to the citizens of this small and sometimes charming city I must apologize, for I vastly prefer its drier and more desolate neighbor, where no cultural museum has ever stood, and certain charming peasants of my acquaintance still ride horses tall and lean and unintelligible (I speak now of both horses and peasants), and are possessed of a sort of hollow-eyed diabolism that can live only in places where people abuse each other in great solitude. But do not rise up in arms against me, noble people of Arkansas, I speak not generally but of a very select minority of my acquaintance, clad utterly in black and burgundy, shimmering like beetles along the dusty roads that may or may not exist at the time of your reading this. Nay friends, chances are you be not these blue haired Achillae, these shadowy and insubstantial folk, for they are spirits congenital to me, and they do not know how to read. Nay Nay, good neighbor, goodly race of giants, burn not down my dwelling on the outskirts of Carlisle: the fulsome and suave ways of the Nephilim have never and never shall come under my scrutiny.

9.

The rice fields that surround Carlisle infuse the air with a unique heady quality that I find intellectually stimulating. My brain, in fact, is humming with activity. Too quickly for me to grasp, it has resolved the issue of my final measuring spoon, and several other household dilemmas, such that I feel a satisfaction and relief. As for the question of my next meal, I remind myself that dinner will be served shortly, and today being Monday the menu had not been announced ahead of time.

I hear dim voices raised outside. I feel along the floor under my couch for an extendible shepherd's crook, with which I am accustomed to opening the french doors to the portico, even though they're twenty feet or so away from me. I find the crook and perform this operation easily, the crook being adapted from a very lightweight metal developed for use in outer space. I immediately regret my curiosity. The sound I heard had come from an intensely ugly peasant, now within sight, and an enormous mosquito the size of a snowball, gorging itself on the blood of that peasant's unfortunate horse, to the pathetic cries of its rider. The mosquito, all the while, emitted a horrific humanoid scream as it sucked from the bleary animal at an astonishing rate. The horse, after a mere moment, began to wobble and sway to the terror of its rider, who clung to the beast even as it finally sank to the earth with an enormous thud. This horse was about ten feet fall, the rider however, a normal sized man, now leapt from the beast and drawing out his six-shooter exploded the pest in a balloon of blood. None of this grotesque display, so silly that I hesitate to describe it, pleased me in the least, and with a few deft flicks of my crook the room was sealed off once again. I mused on the short life of man and beast, on the bloody drama and the unfortunate impossibility of adapting it to the stage, which in turn somewhat devalued the experience for me.

To my intense dismay I soon heard a knock on my front door. I listened to footsteps ascending the grand stairway, and then the tapped signal of my manservant told me that I had a visitor, so I called aloud that he might enter – first making sure that my penis had been put away.

I was struck firstly by my visitor's size. He was in fact extremely small, though of average proportion. From this I deduced that his horse (for he was that same peasant I had seen outside), had been an animal of only normal size.

The man begged my pardon for intruding upon me, but as his horse had just met with a fatal accident, he thought he'd come up "to the big house" as he put it, and ask me for lodging for the evening, as the mosquitos were out and he didn't wish to risk the journey home. I decided to oblige him, and told my servant to show the man to a guest room upstairs.

Before dismissing the horseman, however, I decided to ask him if he had perchance seen five dollars on the ground outside my door. Of course, he had not and answered in the negative, at which I performed a broad dull smile and give him a long blank stare. I pronounced as simply and innocently as I could that we were friends. The peasant seemed pleased by this and was ushered from the room.

After a while a nagging suspicion that I had been struggling with all day became pronounced, namely: my girlfriend was upset. She being absent, I could not immediately verify this, but I took pause to make sure I was at a maximum of remove from any strong emotions that might disturb my equanimity and thus make me unfit to approach her.

Like a man blowing out his candle before sleep, I consciously extinguished my intellectual faculties as well, and felt a tremendous levity invade my body. I foresaw the self-resolution of unknown future events displayed before me, and entertained a mood of nearly theophanic resignation.

10.

Crowding under the leaves at Don Grey's,
your hands were clean so I asked you
to put up my hair. The low rolling slopes of it,
the silver waves
of country stuff. The earth that people believe in
down here is extremely mellow, horny with dust
and lusting after me.

As my red car (spirit) is mounted on the Ferris Wheel
let us remember fondly during its final moments
the town we're living in (Carlisle).
Now we can weep
with the horses who fucking love it here…

***

I was interrupted by two gunshots from downstairs. My brain immediately switched back on, and I felt a horror creep over me, certain that someone had been killed. I sprang from my couch and ran down the stairs in a state of grim expectation. What I discovered in the expansive entryway was my manservant, lying on his back, discharging his now empty handgun at the massive reproduction of Michael Angelo's Sistine Chapel that graces my ceiling.

This monumental reproduction had been painstakingly glued into harmony by a local artisan out of repurposed plastic bags from various stores and restaurants, acquired throughout my travels.

I was astonished, not only to see that my man had shot precisely through God's nipples, but also that blood had begun to trickle from these wounds and splatter the floor below. I remembered that portion of the ceiling roughly corresponded to the guest-room in which my man had only minutes ago escorted our guest. My man explained that the person whom I had believed to be a native Arkansian peasant, now lying dead in my guest room, was in fact...

but my attention had drifted from this good man's story — one that I was certain vindicated him of this murder, completely setting my mind at ease — because just then two sets of doors opened: one to the movie-theatre, from which my girlfriend emerged and stood taking in the scene; the other to the kitchen, where I beheld the chef of my establishment. His hands were still drying themselves on the little towel he kept tucked into his apron string, directly under his proudly protruding belly. He stood with one foot forward, and his head thrown back, exactly like Rodin's great statue of Balzac. He wore an impressive little smile that barely dimpled his cheeks, and I felt, as can only be felt in Arkansas, a clairvoyant message as his brain spoke to mine a fraction of a second before he said aloud the words describing tonight's entrée. Coq au Vin, with rancid butter, accompanied by asparagus soup and Vín de Paille. I nearly crumbled to the blooded tiles at this tremendous news.

PART II: AFTER DINNER

My guest room had been wrecked. In the few minutes that it had been occupied by the fraudulent peasant, its walls had been stripped of their gilt ornate moldings — moldings I had acquired at enormous cost from the Italian villa in which Boccaccio is believed to have written his Decameron. Gone was the little copper piping that snaked through one of the wrecked walls, my silver candlesticks, rugs, a decorative platter that had been borrowed and never returned from a descendant of Pancho Villa, a pair of fine deer-skin gloves — and other sundries were haphazardly jammed into and were poking out from an oversize leather sack.

The two bullets that my man had discharged through the image of God's nipples and through the floor, killing this man from the floor below, had landed miraculously. The dead man had been thrown onto his back on the bed, exposing to us the bullet entry holes, both precisely through his nipples, obliterating them completely.

My manservant quietly left to retrieve some supplies, leaving me with the corpse. I turned his pockets out and did not discover anything besides a tin medallion bearing an image of the Infant of Prague, and five dollars, both of which I slid into my trousers pocket. I could see the top of a tattoo where the collar of the man's shirt lay open, and began unbuttoning his shirt, exposing an increasingly expansive and elaborate tiger's head chest piece. To my astonishment, amid a swirling mess of poorly incorporated objects that somewhat marred and were only half submerged in the image of the tiger, I discovered that the eyes of this beast had been placed directly over…

Now, as I saw the tiger weeping blood, I succumbed to a nervous reaction, one that I am prone to in times of intense stress. I shakily pulled down my pants and squeezed and pulled the shaft of my penis between thumb and forefinger several times until it began to swell, at which I immediately picked up my pants and tucked it away.

The many events of the day were beginning to take their toll on me, and I began to fear that I would be too overworked to perform by the time my girlfriend and I had designated for sexual intercourse.

My manservant entered the room with a cart containing all manner of chemicals and supplies in which I felt a profound disinterest, and I left him to his work with the cadaver. Back on my couch, however, the weeping tiger bothered me. I could not remove the vision of its tearful look and the strange emotion that had been brought to its face by the bullet-holes, and this image blocked out all other sensations. I decided it

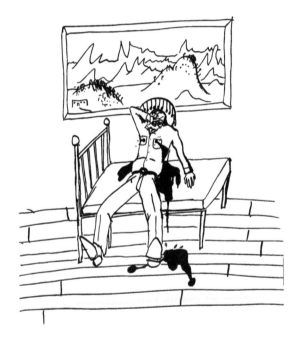

"My guest room had been wrecked."

would be best to return to get a hard look at it, the better to vanquish it from my mind.

I strode back to the room, and found the door already open. To my astonishment, the corpse was gone, as was my manservant and his tools. The blood had been cleaned up and the room was returned to its usual order. Only the bullet-holes in the floor remained to speak of the incident. I decided not to go looking for my man and his burden and instead retired to my room, this time resigned not to leave.

Unfortunately, as I fumbled through my waistcoat pockets, I realized that my fish-fork was missing, and knew immediately that it must have fallen out as I detailed the dead man's body. Thus I found myself once again at the door of the guest room, in the hopes of finding my fork somewhere beneath the bed.

Even worse than before — how I cringe at the thought of relaying this to you, dear reader! — I now beheld a family of ducks, some standing on the floor and some on the bare mattress, none of them interested in my intrusion. I could not fathom how and for what reason they had been put there. My fish-fork was nowhere to be seen, and I began to have a dark foreboding that my fork had made its way into the dead man's clothes. I deplored the silliness of keeping ducks indoors and wracked my brains for some acceptable reason. I hastily retreated to my room.

I pulled several books down from my shelves and flipped listlessly through them, unable to pay the least attention. At last I napped: I napped, I say, because I do not 'sleep.' My rest comes only in short bursts.

I was soon awakened by the clatter of rice trucks on the road nearby, and I listened to their big wooden wheels pass along the dirt road with my eyes closed. After some minutes, when I felt completely at ease and the rumble was become only a distant thing, I picked up my notebook and wrote:

Baseball

I'm here to tell you this is a world of surfing, and we can know even less of others, though they depend so much on my performance, sucking at the gold beneath our skin, milling the flour, catching the fish, that works my body free from the chalk cliff-face.

In this tubercular ward, I reposition myself as if I were the unerring vagina. The truth is terrible, but I'll send you a picture of it at the right price.

Before word of my transformation reached the rotunda,
before the gates to the underworld were jammed
everything seemed to participate
including nature, and its violent twin, real estate. The meaning
of baseball was illuminated on the fields, as the ball was passed
across my forehead.
The game tugged at its rules, unable to detach
 from humidity and the sensation of drowning.

A flaming jewel, the spirit of baseball slipped
from the grasping hands of the ghosts who rule over this realm.

I admit that this poem was something of a surprise to me, as I knew next to nothing about baseball, besides what I had seen many years ago, when I was a Chinese prince borne upon a palanquin to a field in the Catskills. There I beheld to my delight an authentic baseball game. Indeed, that trip would stay with me for many lives, and I recall musing at that time on the game's symbology and its lofty spirit — though I fear I have since lost all taste for actually following the sport.

The time for copulation was nearly upon us, and my girlfriend, presumably in her rooms, was likely bathing herself in anticipation. I felt a strong necessity to dream again, though as I have remarked I only very rarely dream. Nonetheless, I could feel an important dream poking at me from the other side. Valerian, though it had never worked for me in the past, could be acquired. Lemon, applied to the wrist, is said to bring about lucid dreaming, but that would not be helpful or even desirable. Lucid dreaming, long studied as a Buddhist practice, I conceived, was actually a great violence done to the dream, and not by the dreamer but by the waking person. In fact, I disagree with nearly every Buddhist practice down to the least minutia of grammar.

The practice of keeping dream-journals and waking visualizations are of course only further instances of the Buddhist crime against dream.

The only authentic way to induce dreams in a fundamentally non-dreamer, is drugs.

Drugs of course could mean any substance at all, from milk to marijuana to margarine. Since I would be least likely to dream after the extreme relaxation following sexual intercourse, I decided this dream must be made to happen immediately.

After I rang my bell and exchanged a few words with my man, he was quick in bringing me some dried Water Lily flowers, an exquisite onierogen, which I smoked by vaporizing with a small boxy machine connected to a transparent gas-mask attachment. This wonderful flower unfortunately did not also induce sleepiness, so to bring myself over I pulled out and erected my penis (using both hands). This done, my attention drawn away from all earthly worries, I wrapped my penis in a very thin silk cloth imprinted with the circle of the zodiac, and left it out as I reclined on the couch.

PART 3: NIGHT

1

The moonrise over Carlisle was what first bewitched me into settling here, and it is mere luck that the people of this town have not hit upon a strategy to turn this water-influencing meteorite into profit. Contrary to the gawking at "beauty, loveliness," done by my neighbors, I adore this location because here the moon seems more easily destroyed than anywhere else on earth. A sensitive person feels emboldened here, capable of smiting it with ease from the sky. I am among those who hold that the moon is cause of all misfortune on this planet.

It was a bleary, aqueous moon, a waning crescent, that met my vision through the skylight immediately above my bed. After swiftly jerking the covers over my head, I extended my arms to either side in search of my girlfriend, but did not meet with any part of her, save for a sharp hairpin that had apparently come loose during our lovemaking. Without looking I knew this was the hairpin bearing the decorative motif of mating coyotes along its base, which I grasped firmly. Quickly thrusting the pin vertically from my navel, I pierced the thick blanket that covered me.

This blanket had been created from a biblically accurate formula for the creation of The Arc of the Covenant out of animal pelts — though somewhat adapted to the fauna of Carlisle. I peeked above the lip of this immense patchwork of animals and saw that I had pierced the flesh of a porcupine, still bearing its quills, such that my girlfriend's hair-pin mingled with the quills of the animal almost imperceptibly.

My study of the quills and hair-pin vanishing among them, only to reappear as a silver gleam a moment later, threw me into a contemplative mood, and I delighted in watching two similar things show their different materials against each other. Simon Magus, I mused, was said to hold flying demonstrations in which he would with the help of some demon float off of a tall structure designed for that purpose and amaze his onlookers. Simon, a worshipper of uncouth deities, thus provoked the wrath of Christians like Peter who wished to hoard all magic in his own religion. While Simon demonstrated his flight, Peter's fervent prayers caused the demons to abandon Simon, who plummeted to his death. The obvious issue with this story is that it advertises the possibility for an ascent to heaven via the aid of demons. As I watched the oscillations of this hair-pin in and out of visibility, I was struck by the short sightedness of Peter's boast against the power of Simon Magus. One has to wonder if this tale was not a secret lesson invented by Simon Magus himself, to teach adepts in the troubled first century of Christendom. I recall now in my dim youth a tall, thin, darkly bearded man, with somewhat cavernous eyes and hollow cheeks — thought to be very handsome — who introduced himself to me as Simon Magus. He taught me the trick of stealing a bicycle by removing the front wheel, if that had been the only place by which the bike was locked, and riding away using only the remaining wheel.

I noticed that my genitals were in a state of perfect equilibrium. They were neither wet nor dry, but fleshy and rubbery, neither aroused nor quite forgotten. They buzzed with a secret intelligence. I pulled the blanket over my head again, and after moving my genitals around in a fit of haphazard delights, I closed my eyes and lay still.

2.

But sleep did not come to me. I felt the maleficent influence of the moon weighing on me where it shone down in a rectangle from the skylight precisely over my body. Though the animal skins kept some of its effects at bay, they could do nothing to shield me from its weight, and while in the past I have often found that added pressure to be comforting and sleep inducing, it only annoyed me and my scalp began to itch. Having first pulled my girlfriend's hairpin back through the blanket, I slid several feet to my right. No longer directly under the moon's rays, the blanket felt light and airy above me. Very likely I was under a patch of raccoons. I should add that my bed is the repurposed coal-room of a steam engine, its sides sheared off. Thus my bed is unusually wide and hence my need for an Arc of the Covenant sized blanket.

By moving over as I'd done, I had repositioned myself between two mattresses. I began to squeeze myself into the crevice between them, which easily opened for me as the mattresses slid aside on railings at the head and foot-boards to permit my passage. As I descended, I felt great pleasure from the thought that Simon Magus has existed for all of recorded history and that he should pass on some tidbit of wisdom to me.

As I lay on the floor beneath my bed, I rummaged in the pockets of my night clothes, and recovered therefrom a small obsidian marble, which I let roll from my hand. I then turned and followed it by ear in the darkness until it reached the exact center of my very gently sloping room. Once the ball stopped I groped around its vicinity and soon found a rope pull, which released a small trap door while simultaneously dropping a rope ladder which ended directly above my favorite couch where I had spent most of the day. I was not, however, interested in returning to my day-room, and instead took advantage of the light from below to squint into the darkness beneath my bed.

A few feet away, no bigger than a cigar, lay what I knew to be a mummified snake. First making sure to reload the rope-ladder and close the trap, I proceeded toward the mummy. Then, once the snake was in my hand (and I had offered a blessing to the Fire Serpent by pretending to breast feed it), I had only a few more feet to crawl before I reached the end of my bed.

3.

Once I pushed aside the black velvet bed skirt and stood in the indirect illumination of the skylight, I held the mummified snake to my lips. I lightly passed it across them and felt its thin papyrus wrapping. Like many times before, I nearly succumbed to the urge to dunk the dehydrated creature and his wrappings into a tall carafe of water I keep on a dresser that stood before me; but I mastered this great temptation and contented myself by merely licking his wrapper with the tip of my tongue. I then prepared to deposit him in my uppermost dresser drawer, reserved generally for socks and underwear and small objects.

Upon opening the drawer, however, I lost all thought of depositing him there, because my drawer had been emptied of my usual undergarments and sundries, and I discovered a mere void with the exception of some buttons and screws. While I had originally assumed the unusual location of my snake-mummy to be a mere accident of housekeeping, I now suspected responsibility lay with whoever had absconded with the things in my drawer. This filled me with a sudden dread, and in a few swift bounds I traversed the room to a tall ebony cabinet. This cabinet had been fashioned from infinite small wooden toys — ground down and carefully glued together. I cranked the handle and heaved a great sigh of relief — it remained locked. Clearly then, this strange crime against me had not been for any common gain, for in that cabinet I keep the solid gold figurines that represent my grandmother at significant moments of her life, many of them sizable, as she had at times been astonishingly rotund.

I began to feel some trepidation as to what I might do with my mummy, which I realized I was squeezing in my inadvertently clenched fist. Once I'd shuffled him in and out of different pockets I decided to nestle him — after first pinching my penis a few times so it began to stiffen — in my underwear alongside my member.

4.

My night-clothes are manufactured from several Victorian dresses, pulled apart and remade into a suitably male garment of pants, shirt, and vest.

The overall effect of this suit — sleek and black with delicate embroidery — is suggestive of a Spanish grandee. I am aware that this guise creates terror in those who without warning should see me wearing it at night.

I felt restless, and while considering whether or not to return to my bed or perhaps ring my manservant for a bit of conversation, I relieved my nervous tension by pulling at my testicles, gingerly, with my fingertips and nails, so as not to disturb the snake-mummy that ran alongside my penis and fell overtop of them. At this very intimate moment I heard coyotes screaming in the field, and wondered if the dead horse beneath my portico had been removed, or if it would now be prey for these animals and other such that nibble corpses.

I reached my hand up to the top of the cabinet and brought down a tall thin ledger-book, with a golf pencil clipped to the cover which doubled as a clipboard. After fishing a thumb-sized flashlight from my pocket and placing it between my teeth, I wrote this poem:

Sit down in my astral chair,
inside the outside of the sky
and hear the screen door rumble
on its virtuous track, the total person.

We can hide out here all night,
and after that we'll be murderers
officially, like a villanelle
hardening the hearts of things
forcing them to sit with us,

though there is no moon real enough
to swing a garland of seagulls at, one is enslaved
to the purport of the senses,
and the being that disorients them. The night sky
is full of lassos of every kind of substance: be kind to
them. Here is every kind of sustenance, though one feels
conceptually to have passed across them, to bear
the howling mint of ducklessness… but do not let
the little geniuses distract you from breathing
onto the heart's false mirror. Aprender,
to learn, perhaps this time, cryptic hot shampoo.

The poem overall had a pleasing gait and I found it to be more intellectually inclined than usual. I suspect that an analytical part of my brain has been overstimulated by the mystery of my missing and misplaced things.

5.

I replaced my ledger-book atop the cabinet, feeling somewhat more at ease having gained insight into my mental state, but then took the book to hand again feeling that I would want it momentarily.

In order to combat my feeble attempts at demystifying recent occurrences, I felt it best to retrace my steps by removing the snake-mummy from my underwear which might possibly have been a step toward rationalization (though obviously much disguised).

This little setback brought with it a stream of incoherent emotions, but I was careful not to blame myself, for that alone would have been an ethical failure, whereas my perceived 'setback' was not any different in value than any other event — indeed, this setback and its rectification were held in a centrifugal grip of iron, and I waded carefully through all manner of psychological feints and self-deceits such as inevitably arise with value judgements.

In recognition of my overwrought state, I rang for my manservant by way of a pull-rope next to the door that swung a bell in the servant's quarters. My man appeared almost immediately, dressed in fresh clothes and shaved, I noted. I communicated to him my desire for a strong kava-kava beverage, which it is my habit to drink at all hours.

I recalled the rumor among some that kava causes short-term impotence, and I smiled in the darkness, while tugging my penis appreciatively, for kava had quite the opposite effect on me. As I erected myself, images of my girlfriend appeared before my mind's eye. I beheld her in a series of positions suggestive of kundalini, the object of which is to excite a woman in such a way as to harvest her undesecrated astral essence, which physical fluid is caught on a leaf or in a cup and then consumed. The positions before me however varied immensely from those traditional to kundalini; they were as far removed as possible, it would seem, as if I were considering only the most distant branches of possible relation. The thought of my girlfriend dressed as a schoolteacher-cum-nanny goat, or of her copulating with a cone of sugar — only two of the images that revolved in my mind — filled me with pride and respect for her. One particularly touching image of lesbianism brought me nearly to tears of happiness.

As these images gradually faded, a sentence began to compose itself in my mind:

Conosco el niño es la tomata giganta para mi pregunta.

This struck me as a sign of affirmation, and increased my feeling of already profound joyfulness.

6.

My man entered with a silver serving tray bearing some vigorously mixed kava, still swirling in its glass. This I grasped and gulped down — kava is an unpleasant tasting beverage. I replaced the glass onto my man's tray and he retreated with a backwards leap through the open door, closing it behind him with the agility of a sphinx.

Then, to my intense excitement, I remembered my dream from earlier in the day, shortly before making love with my girlfriend. Though brief, this dream struck me as profound and of very fine quality.

Impossibly large heaps of packed snow, larger than houses, are falling as if they'd been dumped from the sky. These fall only in the distance, plopping onto the mountains, crushing trees and shrubs, but they do not overly worry me. Suddenly, however, a nearby hill is smothered by one of these immense heaps, which sends boulders of snow exploding towards me. These I barely dodge as further massive bombardments follow, landing all around me. I plunge into my cabin to discover my disconcertingly calm family assembled all in a row facing me. This was not, however, my real family, and in the dream I was struck by their generalized quality. My plain and unintelligent looking sisters are dressed warmly and stand next to each other at my gaunt old granny's shoulder. Granny sits in dirty clothes and an apron, holding a shotgun across her knees. She gestures with her hand, grimly summoning me.

Of immediate importance is the way in which this dream prefigures my overexcitement at the loss of my clothes, in the various bombardments that represent anxiety. My grim family in their silence represents the kava I've just taken, its bitter and alcoholic taste.

Had I remembered this dream only moments earlier, might I not have been in control of my fate?

7.

As I replaced my ledger-book I discovered that I had neglected to put my penis away, and I unceremoniously thrust it back into my pants. As

I did so I recalled an old hallucination that I had had in my youth: while I sat in an auditorium I saw a dirty pigeon flap noisily over my head, showering feathers onto the audience. I found comfort in this memory of a liminal bird, which is as an anchor to me now in the storm of unpredictability surrounding the exposure of my penis.

I stood for some time with my eyes closed taking deep breaths, holding them in and breathing them out through my nose. I've always suffered from a nagging remembrance of someone telling me how one should breathe in through their nose (or mouth), and out through the other, though I could never remember which. Nor do I care, but this person's didactic offering lodged itself in my young and vulnerable brain, and I live with it now as with a catch in my breath, criticizing my most intimate and supposedly automatic function.

There is no religion without its mystery of breath. Buddhism, however, stands out for its particular obsession with mediating respiration. Admittedly some practices are effective, but the politics are dubious — even frightening. Second worst in this regard is Swedenborgianism.

A tingling numbness began to torment my left hand. I shook it vigorously but to no effect. I then straightened my fingers and slid my hand into my rear pants pocket as if it were a holster, before collapsing in this awkward position onto the ground in a total loss of limb-function.

8.

On the floor, I lay immobile. I realized my good fortune in that if I had not put them away mere moments ago my genitals would have been exposed in this compromising position. From my vantage I could see little besides the velvet bedskirt. This bedskirt like all fine velvet, is made of silk. This silk however came from many unraveled kimonos, most of great antiquity. The smell this silk exudes is fresh and sweet with something panther-like about it.

Also within my sight, I descried a small metal figurine of the Chrysler Building. Like much in New York, it had little to no value in situ, but once removed it was as good as legal tender, especially in Arkansas, and particularly among the younger set, to whom New York is virtually unknown except as a place of myth and legend, a voluminous cloud of precision and excellence and fame and glory. Ah, to live and die in New York! Living would count for something, if it were to be a part of the great golden machine of man's wondrous progress and industry, the genius of civilization! Alas, like all peasants, they don't know what they have.

I let my eyes roam across the many little windows of this famous building and its 77 brick floors, briefly the tallest building in the world.

This giant architectural achievement sadly was of no use to me at this time. I imagined the miniature lightening rod atop the statue sawing through the invisible ropes that had suddenly bound me. This did in fact improve upon my condition, and as I felt some mobility return to me I was able to pivot my body in such a way as to free my hand from my pocket. That, however, was as much as I could do.

The slight readjustment afforded me a view of certain other objects of great interest.

Closest to me was a small pile of books: Agatha Christie, the Gnostic Gospels, The Debauched Hospodar, The New Justine, a thick roadmap of the mid-west, Quaint Customs and Manners of Japan. It was not this that interested me, but atop the pile I could just barely discern the form of a juvenile swordfish, no more than five inches in length, the skeleton of which I had had preserved in transparent resin. With this skeleton fully occupying my mind, I imagined its sharp sword-like skull slashing through a gordian knot of ropes, chains, and restraints. Feeling immediately rushed back into my body, and I heard a horrific male scream precede from around me and vanish out through the skylight. Gradually I regained my feet. What I had not noticed is that I stood directly in the middle of a white chalk circle drawn with various figures surrounding it, and in the center a curious sigil — though now smudged beyond recognition — where my body had fallen. The circle had been cut in several places, presumably by my efforts. I nearly began to seek some reason for the event...

In order to rid my mind of thoughts I contemplated masturbating, but I felt exhausted and still fragile in my regained strength. I contented myself with scattering the chalk circle and its various signs by slowly shuffling around its perimeter. While I did this I mentally composed the following poem.

The ruinous rains come four times a year

and furthermore a man will invariably trace a squiggly
        spine
on the wall and it turns out I'm looking at me.

With the swords that wiggle out from a blue film
and cut out the shape of an arrow:

with what I call 'substance abuse.'
The Poet said, to his beloved:

I'm sorry, I have the wrong information.

'With the swords that wiggle out from a blue film' seems to be a celebration of my release from bondage by the aid of the swordfish, which had a bluish color when it retained its flesh. My mention of blue film also suggests the blue sky opposite that of night, the moonless sky of day, of salvation, the salvific item and from whence it had come.

The rest of the poem strikes me as a boring expression of familiar themes. However, that does not mean it's bad per se. I don't even know what's familiar until it's written, and then just as quickly it's gone. Rather than the dullness I feel it possesses now, it may become instructive once it's thoroughly forgotten. For this reason, I retrieved my ledger book and recorded the poem for my later consideration.

9.

I began to recall that while I was incapacitated in the magic circle, I received a stream of information, somewhat like a dream, but with the feeling that it had happened elsewhere, outside of my body.

This information described my struggle against two creatures in the form of a young couple that ghoulishly harassed and at times murdered members of a crowd of people locked in a bowling alley. After a great struggle, I was able to wrest from them a highly unusual weapon that shot a kind of sticky pink goo. With this in hand I went on the hunt, but I was unable to locate our persecutors. A bystander to whom I had called out informed me that I had grown a large ornate black aura. This looked somewhat like Victorian lace. I quickly turned around and shot my aura with the goo gun, but it had no effect, leaving my aura in place and dripping with goo, giving it the appearance of wrought iron.

I could recall dimly many other streams of information that I had received simultaneously without cognizing, none of them necessarily related to each-other except that they formed a single standing wave, each particle remaining distinct, as if the matrix that contained these stories had been filled in radically by innumerable passing voices. One might compare the effect to a chance-produced library stored within the very material of a seashell.

10.

I could see by the altered quality of the light that dawn had nearly arrived. With my penis becoming suddenly erect, I assumed a position of prayer. Kneeling with my elbows on my bed and hands clasped before my face, I did not address any prayers but focused all of my attention on my body, which is clearly what this posture was designed for. By slight adjustments of my hips, waist, and thighs, imperceptible to a spectator, and by subtle changes in my breathing which I altered as I saw fit, I was able to bring myself to climax.

Of even greater interest, I was able to retain my emission within my body by using a subtle muscle group that I discovered to be accessible only at this hour. This emission, reabsorbed, would satisfy my craving for stimulants throughout the day.

fin.

The author wishes to thank Haley Paul,
Billie Chernicoff, Carlos Lara,
and Joel Newberger.

Other Authors of NEW BOOKS &
NEW SMUT SERIES:

Maggie Zavgren
Nolan J. Bibb
Jonny Collazo
Losarc Raal
Joel Newberger
Lila Dunlap
Douglas Piccinnini
and others…